Cytomegalovirus Infection Demystified

A Comprehensive and Practical Approach to Understanding Symptoms, Causes, Treatments and Conquering the Condition

| Things You Must Know |

Isabella White

About the Book

Cytomegalovirus Infection Demystified is an essential guide for anyone looking to understand this pervasive yet often misunderstood condition better. With its comprehensive coverage of CMV, including its potential impact, management strategies, and preventative measures, this book is an authoritative resource that can help you stay informed and take control of your health. Whether you are a healthcare professional, a patient, or someone interested in learning about CMV, ***Cytomegalovirus Infection Demystified*** is a must-read.

White's meticulous research and accessible writing style make this book an invaluable resource for those living with CMV, their families, healthcare providers, and anyone interested in public health. The book's detailed chapters cover everything from the basic biology of the virus to the latest advancements in treatment and the ongoing search for a vaccine.

Combining scientific precision and empathetic storytelling, ***Cytomegalovirus Infection Demystified*** enlightens and reassures individuals impacted by CMV, providing them with comfort and optimism. It is a testament to patients' resilience and the medical community's dedication to combating this silent threat.

Whether you are a medical professional, a patient, or someone seeking to expand your knowledge, this book will be a crucial tool in your arsenal against CMV. Join Isabella White on a journey of discovery and empowerment with ***Cytomegalovirus Infection Demystified.***

About the Author

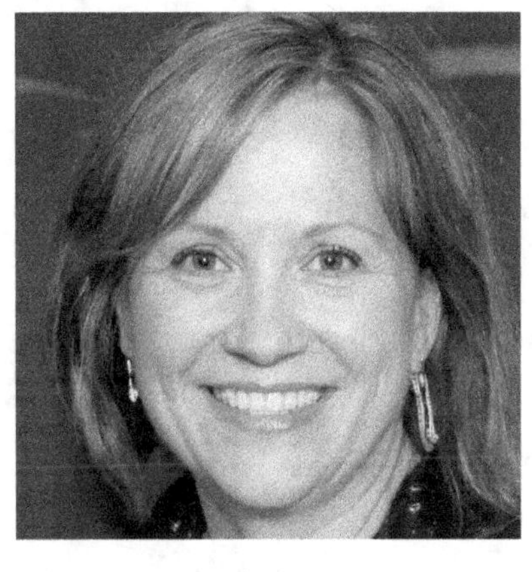

Isabella White brings profound expertise and compassion to illuminating health challenges through her writing. As a integrative medicine practitioner, she blends conventional medical knowledge with evidence-based holistic approaches.

Dr. White received her medical degree and a master's in traditional Chinese medicine from the University of Washington. She has over 15 years of clinical experience, empowering patients to optimize their health and well-being.

As a seasoned health writer, Dr. White is renowned for distilling complex medical concepts into accessible, engaging language. She has published articles on integrative techniques in medical journals and books.

With over a decade immersed in research and education, Dr. White offers readers scientifically rigorous yet humanistic insights. Her clinical experience and her appreciation for patient perspectives make her writing resonate with diverse audiences.

Dr. White aims to equip readers with the tools needed to secure optimal care and outcomes by explaining health topics with wisdom, empathy, and sensitivity. She brings clarity, reassurance, and hope grounded in science and compassion.

Table of Contents

Introduction

Cytomegalovirus (CMV) is a widespread viral infection from the herpes virus family. It's common and often asymptomatic, meaning many contract it without realizing it. However, for certain individuals, such as those with weakened immune systems or pregnant women, CMV can pose serious health risks.

The prevalence of CMV is staggering, with estimates suggesting that between 50% and 80% of adults in the United States have been infected with the virus by the time they reach 40 years of age. While most healthy individuals who contract CMV experience no symptoms or only mild, flu-like symptoms, the virus can have severe consequences for specific groups.

For individuals with compromised immune systems, such as those undergoing organ transplants, receiving cancer treatments, or living with HIV/AIDS, CMV can cause life-threatening complications. In these cases, the virus can lead to severe infections affecting various organs, including the lungs, liver, brain, and eyes.

Pregnant women who contract CMV for the first time during pregnancy can potentially pass the infection on to their unborn child, a condition known as congenital CMV. This can result in devastating congenital disabilities, including hearing loss, vision impairment, intellectual disabilities, and even stillbirth or miscarriage.

Despite its prevalence and potential risks, many people remain unaware of CMV or underestimate its impact. This lack of awareness often leads to inadequate preventive measures, delayed diagnosis, and suboptimal management of the infection and its consequences.

The Importance of Awareness and Education

Raising awareness and promoting cytomegalovirus (CMV) education is crucial for several reasons. First and foremost, it helps individuals understand the potential risks and impacts of the infection, particularly those with weakened immune systems or pregnant women.

Many people are unaware of the dangers of cytomegalovirus (CMV) and assume it is a harmless virus with no significant consequences. This can lead to a false sense of security and result in a failure to take necessary precautions or seek timely medical attention. It's crucial to understand that this misconception can have severe consequences, and we must educate ourselves on the risks associated with CMV.

Furthermore, limited knowledge about CMV can contribute to delayed diagnosis and inadequate management of the infection. Healthcare professionals may overlook or misdiagnose CMV-related symptoms, leading to missed opportunities for early intervention and treatment.

Education and awareness also play a vital role in preventing the spread of CMV. By understanding the modes of transmission and implementing appropriate hygiene practices, individuals can reduce the risk of contracting or transmitting the virus to vulnerable populations, such as newborns and immunocompromised individuals.

Increased awareness and education can also facilitate open discussions about CMV, breaking down stigmas and misconceptions that may exist around the infection. This open dialogue can encourage individuals to seek support, share their experiences, and contribute to a more comprehensive understanding of the condition.

Moreover, raising awareness can drive research efforts and funding opportunities to develop better diagnostic methods, treatments, and preventive measures against CMV. As more people become informed about the potential consequences of the infection, there will be increased demand for effective solutions and support for scientific endeavors in this area.

This book aims to promote awareness and education about CMV by empowering individuals with knowledge and understanding. It enables readers to make informed decisions, seek appropriate medical care, and implement preventive measures to protect themselves and their loved ones from the potential risks associated with this widespread viral infection.

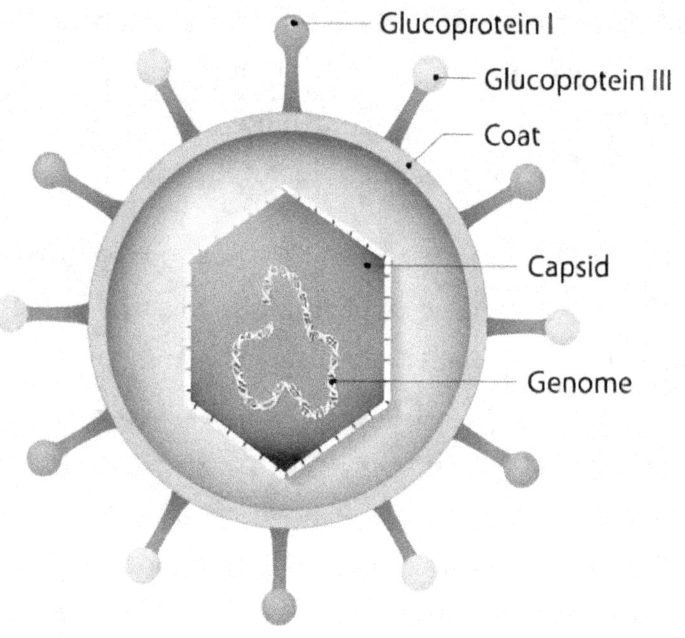

Chapter 1

THE BASICS OF CYTOMEGALOVIRUS

What is Cytomegalovirus?

Cytomegalovirus (CMV) is a member of the herpes virus family, a group of viruses known for establishing lifelong infections in the human body. Unlike other well-known herpes viruses, such as the ones that cause cold sores or chickenpox, CMV primarily targets specific cells and tissues within the body rather than causing widespread skin infections.

At its core, CMV is a complex and highly adaptive virus that has evolved alongside humans for centuries. It is adept at evading the body's immune defenses, allowing it to persist in a dormant state within cells for extended periods without causing noticeable symptoms. This ability to remain undetected is one of the reasons why CMV infections are so widespread, with a significant portion of the global population carrying the virus without even realizing it.

Despite its stealthy nature, CMV is not always harmless. In individuals with weakened immune systems, such as those undergoing organ transplants, receiving cancer treatments, or living with HIV/AIDS, the virus can reactivate and cause severe complications affecting various organs, including the lungs, liver, brain, and eyes. Additionally, pregnant women who contract a primary CMV infection during pregnancy can potentially pass the virus on to their unborn child, leading to congenital CMV. This condition can result in severe congenital disabilities and long-term developmental disabilities.

While CMV is primarily known for its impact on vulnerable populations, it is important to note that even healthy individuals can experience mild to moderate symptoms when initially infected with the virus. These symptoms can range from fatigue and fever to swollen glands and a sore throat, often mimicking those of other common viral infections like the flu or mononucleosis.

It is crucial for individuals, healthcare professionals, and public health authorities to understand the nature of CMV, its modes of transmission, and its potential to cause harm in specific circumstances. By demystifying this complex virus and raising awareness about its existence and potential consequences, we can prevent its spread, manage its impact, and ultimately conquer the challenges of this persistent and adaptable infection.

Historical Perspective

The history of cytomegalovirus (CMV) is an intriguing tale that spans centuries, intertwining with major scientific discoveries and medical advancements. While the virus likely coexisted with humans for thousands of years, its formal identification and understanding have evolved, reflecting the progression of medical knowledge and technological capabilities.

The earliest known reference to CMV can be traced back to the late 19th century, when two German pathologists, Hugo Ribbert and Johann Ritter von Rittershain, independently observed abnormally large cells in the lungs and kidneys of stillborn infants. These enlarged cells, later named "cytomegalic" cells, were the first clues to the existence of an unknown pathogen.

Significant breakthroughs in CMV research occurred in the 1950s. In 1954, Margaret Gladys Smith, a virologist at the Viral and Rickettsial Disease Laboratory in Boston, successfully isolated and cultivated the virus from two cases involving infants with congenital cytomegalic inclusion disease. This groundbreaking achievement paved the way for further investigations into the nature and behavior of the virus.

Throughout the following decades, researchers worldwide devoted substantial efforts to unraveling the mysteries of CMV. Advancements in molecular biology, immunology, and diagnostic technologies played a crucial role in deepening our understanding of the virus's structure, modes of transmission, and its ability to evade the human immune system.

One of the most significant milestones in CMV research came in the 1980s, when the virus was recognized as a major cause of life-threatening infections in individuals with weakened immune systems, particularly those undergoing organ transplants or living with HIV/AIDS. This realization highlighted the urgent need for effective antiviral treatments and preventive measures to protect these vulnerable populations.

Today, CMV remains a subject of intense scientific investigation, with ongoing research focused on developing improved diagnostic tools, more effective antiviral therapies, and potential vaccine candidates. These days, many people have access to very advanced molecular techniques that have helped us learn a lot about how CMV affects and changes the human immune system. This has helped us understand this challenging and complicated virus even better.

Prevalence and Epidemiology

Cytomegalovirus (CMV) is one of the most prevalent viral infections worldwide, affecting individuals across all geographic regions, socioeconomic levels, and age groups. The prevalence and epidemiology of CMV are striking, reflecting the virus's ability to spread efficiently and establish lifelong infections within the human body.

Globally, over half of the world's population is estimated to carry CMV, with seroprevalence rates (the presence of antibodies indicating past exposure) ranging from 45% to 100% in different countries and populations. In developed nations like the United States and Western Europe, seroprevalence rates typically range from 50% to 80% among adults, increasing with age.

However, the prevalence of CMV is generally higher in developing countries and regions with lower socioeconomic status, where factors such as overcrowding, poor sanitation, and limited access to healthcare can contribute to more rapid transmission. In some parts of Africa, Asia, and

Latin America, seroprevalence rates can exceed 90% in certain population groups.

Interestingly, CMV prevalence also varies based on specific demographic characteristics. Women tend to have higher seroprevalence rates than men, likely due to increased exposure through childcare and caregiving responsibilities. Additionally, individuals from lower socioeconomic backgrounds and those living in crowded living conditions are at greater risk of contracting CMV due to more frequent exposure to the virus through close contact and shared environments.

The modes of transmission for CMV are diverse, contributing to its widespread nature. The virus can be transmitted through bodily fluids, such as saliva, urine, blood, and breast milk, as well as through close personal contact, sexual activity, and vertical transmission from mother to child during pregnancy or childbirth. This multitude of transmission routes makes it challenging to completely prevent exposure, particularly in populations with highly prevalent CMV.

While CMV infections are generally asymptomatic or cause mild symptoms in healthy individuals, the virus can pose significant risks to certain vulnerable populations. Congenital CMV, which occurs when the virus is transmitted from an infected mother to her unborn child, is a leading cause of congenital disabilities and developmental disabilities worldwide. Additionally, CMV is a significant threat to individuals with weakened immune systems, such as organ transplant recipients, cancer patients undergoing chemotherapy, and those living with HIV/AIDS.

Understanding the prevalence and epidemiology of CMV is crucial for developing effective public health strategies, implementing preventive measures, and prioritizing research efforts to address the challenges posed by this widespread viral infection. By recognizing the global burden of CMV and its potential impact, we can better allocate resources and tailor interventions to protect the most vulnerable populations.

Chapter 2

TRANSMISSION AND RISK FACTORS

How CMV is Spread

Cytomegalovirus (CMV) is a highly contagious virus that can be transmitted through various routes, making it a widespread and persistent infection. Understanding the different modes of transmission is crucial for implementing effective preventive measures and protecting vulnerable populations from the potential consequences of CMV.

One of the primary ways CMV is spread is through direct contact with bodily fluids, such as saliva, urine, blood, semen, and breast milk, of an infected individual. This can occur through activities like kissing, sharing utensils or drinking containers, sexual contact, or exposure to infectious secretions during childbirth or breastfeeding.

CMV can also be transmitted through close personal contact, particularly in settings where individuals live or work in close proximity. This transmission mode is especially relevant in daycare centers, schools, and long-term care facilities, where the virus can easily spread through shared toys, surfaces, or caregiving activities.

Another significant route of CMV transmission is vertical transmission, which occurs when an infected mother passes the virus to her unborn child during pregnancy or to the newborn during delivery. This type of transmission can lead to congenital CMV. This condition can cause severe congenital disabilities and long-term developmental disabilities in the affected child.

In addition to these routes, CMV can also be transmitted through organ transplantation or blood transfusions. However, rigorous screening and safety measures have significantly reduced the risk of transmission through these means in many developed countries.

It's important to note that individuals with weakened immune systems, such as organ transplant recipients, individuals undergoing cancer treatment, or those living with HIV/AIDS, are at a higher risk of acquiring CMV or experiencing reactivation of a previously dormant infection. In these cases, the virus can cause severe and life-threatening complications affecting various organs and systems.

High-Risk Populations

While cytomegalovirus (CMV) infections are generally asymptomatic or cause mild symptoms in healthy individuals, certain populations are at an increased risk of developing severe complications from the virus. Understanding these high-risk groups is crucial for implementing targeted preventive measures and ensuring appropriate medical care.

1. **Infants with Congenital CMV:**

   Congenital CMV, which occurs when the virus is transmitted from an infected mother to her unborn child during pregnancy, is one of the most significant risk factors. Infants born with congenital CMV are at risk of developing a range of congenital disabilities and long-term disabilities, including hearing loss, vision impairment, intellectual disabilities, and developmental delays. Early identification and treatment are crucial for minimizing the potential impact on these infants.

2. **Individuals with Weak Immune Systems:**

   People with compromised immune systems are at a higher risk of developing severe CMV infections. This includes organ transplant recipients, individuals undergoing cancer treatment (particularly those receiving stem cell or bone marrow transplants), and those living with HIV/AIDS. In these cases, CMV can reactivate from a previously dormant state and cause life-threatening complications affecting various organs, such as pneumonia, gastrointestinal disease, and retinitis (an infection of the retina that can lead to vision loss).

3. **Premature Infants:**

Premature infants, particularly those born before 32 weeks of gestation or with very low birth weights, are at an increased risk of developing severe CMV infections. Their immature immune systems and prolonged hospital stays make them more susceptible to acquiring the virus, which can lead to severe complications like pneumonia, hepatitis, and neurological problems.

4. **Healthcare Workers:**

Healthcare professionals, especially those working in settings with a high prevalence of CMV, such as neonatal or transplant units, are at an elevated risk of occupational exposure to the virus. Proper preventive measures, including personal protective equipment and adherence to infection control protocols, are essential for minimizing the risk of transmission.

5. **Individuals in Close Contact Settings:** CMV can spread rapidly in environments where people live or work close together, such as daycare centers, schools, long-term care facilities, and military barracks. Children and caregivers in these settings are at a higher risk of contracting the virus due to the increased likelihood of exposure to bodily fluids and close personal contact.

Identifying and understanding these high-risk populations is vital for implementing targeted prevention strategies, such as promoting awareness, practicing good hygiene, and adhering to infection control protocols. Additionally, early diagnosis and appropriate medical management are crucial for minimizing the potential complications and long-term consequences of CMV infections in these vulnerable groups.

Preventative Measures

Preventing the transmission of cytomegalovirus (CMV) is crucial, especially for protecting high-risk populations from the potential consequences of the infection. While complete eradication of CMV may not be feasible due to its widespread nature, various preventive measures can significantly reduce the risk of transmission and minimize the impact of the virus.

- **Practicing Good Hygiene:** Maintaining proper hand hygiene is one of the most effective measures against the spread of CMV. It is crucial to frequently wash your hands with soap and water, especially after handling bodily fluids, changing diapers, or coming into contact with potentially contaminated surfaces. To minimize the risk of transmission, it is also advisable to cover your coughs and sneezes, avoid sharing personal items like utensils or drinking containers, and keep the environment clean.

- **Implementing Infection Control Measures:**
  In healthcare settings, strict adherence to infection control protocols is vital for preventing the spread of CMV. This includes using personal protective equipment (PPE) when handling bodily fluids, proper disinfection and sterilization of medical equipment, and following standard precautions for patient care.

- **Screening and Testing:**
  Regular screening and testing for CMV can help identify infected individuals, especially in high-risk populations such as pregnant women, organ and stem cell transplant recipients, and individuals with compromised immune systems. Early detection allows prompt intervention and treatment, reducing the risk of severe complications.

- **Safe Handling of Blood and Bodily Fluids:**
  Ensuring the safety of blood products and other bodily fluids is crucial to preventing

CMV transmission. Blood banks and healthcare facilities should implement rigorous screening measures and follow strict protocols for handling and processing blood and blood products to minimize the risk of CMV transmission through transfusions or organ transplantation.

- **Prenatal Care and Education:**
  For pregnant women, receiving regular prenatal care and education about CMV is essential. Healthcare providers should discuss the risks of CMV during pregnancy, recommend appropriate precautions (such as avoiding contact with bodily fluids from young children), and offer screening and counseling services to expectant mothers.

- **Vaccine Development:**
  While no licensed CMV vaccine is available, ongoing research focuses on developing safe and effective vaccines to prevent CMV infections, particularly in high-risk populations. Successful vaccine development could significantly reduce the burden of CMV

and protect vulnerable individuals from the potential consequences of the infection.

Implementing a combination of these preventive measures tailored to specific high-risk populations and settings can significantly reduce the risk of CMV transmission and minimize the potential impact of the virus. Through a comprehensive approach that emphasizes education, hygiene, infection control, and targeted interventions, we can work towards conquering the challenges of this widespread viral infection.

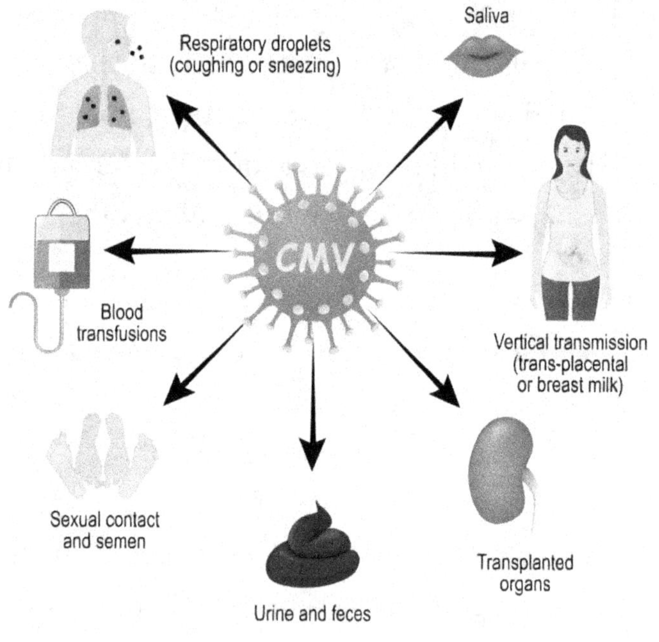

Chapter 3

SIGNS AND SYMPTOMS

Recognizing CMV Infection

Cytomegalovirus (CMV) is often referred to as a "silent" or "stealth" virus because many individuals who contract the infection experience no symptoms or only mild, nonspecific symptoms that can easily be mistaken for other common illnesses. However, recognizing the potential signs and symptoms of CMV infection is crucial, especially for individuals in high-risk groups, as it can aid in early diagnosis and prompt treatment, potentially preventing severe complications.

In healthy individuals with a robust immune system, the initial CMV infection, known as the primary infection, may present with flu-like symptoms such as:

1. Fatigue and weakness
2. Fever
3. Sore throat
4. Muscle aches
5. Swollen lymph nodes

These symptoms are generally mild and may go unnoticed or be attributed to other viral infections. However, in some cases, the primary CMV infection can cause more severe symptoms, including a mononucleosis-like illness with prolonged fever, extreme fatigue, and an enlarged spleen or liver.

It's important to note that after the initial infection, CMV becomes latent, meaning it remains dormant in the body without causing any symptoms. However, in individuals with weakened immune systems, such as organ transplant recipients, those undergoing cancer treatment, or individuals living with HIV/AIDS, the latent CMV can reactivate and cause significant complications.

Symptoms of CMV reactivation or severe infection in immunocompromised individuals can vary depending on the organ system affected but may include:

1. **Pneumonia:** Cough, shortness of breath, and fever
2. **Gastrointestinal disease:** Abdominal pain, diarrhea, and nausea
3. **Retinitis:** Vision problems, floaters, and potentially vision loss
4. **Hepatitis:** Yellowing of the skin and eyes, abdominal pain, and fatigue
5. **Encephalitis:** Headache, confusion, seizures, and neurological deficits

In newborns with congenital CMV (acquired from their mothers during pregnancy), the symptoms can be devastating and may include:

1. Premature birth
2. Small size for gestational age
3. Jaundice
4. Rash or purple skin discoloration
5. Hearing loss

6. Vision problems

7. Developmental delays or intellectual disabilities

While many CMV infections may be asymptomatic or present with mild, nonspecific symptoms, it is crucial to know the potential signs and seek medical attention, especially for individuals in high-risk groups or those experiencing persistent or severe symptoms. Early recognition and diagnosis can significantly improve CMV infection management and outcomes, preventing potential complications and protecting the health of vulnerable populations.

Symptoms in Different Demographics

Cytomegalovirus (CMV) can affect individuals of all ages and demographics; however, the symptoms and severity of the infection can vary significantly depending on the individual's age, immune status, and overall health. Understanding how CMV presents in different demographic groups is crucial for early recognition, accurate diagnosis, and appropriate management.

- **Newborns and Infants:**
  Congenital CMV, which occurs when the virus is transmitted from an infected mother to her unborn child during pregnancy, can have devastating consequences for newborns and infants. Symptoms may include premature birth, low birth weight, jaundice, hepatosplenomegaly (enlarged liver and spleen), petechial rash, pneumonitis, and neurological abnormalities such as microcephaly, cerebral calcifications, and sensorineural hearing loss.

- **Children and Adolescents:**
  In healthy children and adolescents with a robust immune system, primary CMV infection is often asymptomatic or may present with mild, nonspecific symptoms such as fever, fatigue, sore throat, and swollen lymph nodes. However, some children may develop a mononucleosis-like illness with prolonged fever, extreme fatigue, and hepatosplenomegaly.

- **Healthy Adults:**

  In healthy adults with a competent immune system, a primary CMV infection may cause mild flu-like symptoms, including fever, fatigue, a sore throat, and swollen lymph nodes. However, many individuals may experience no symptoms or attribute the mild symptoms to other common viral illnesses.

- **Pregnant Women:**

  For pregnant women who contract a primary CMV infection during pregnancy, the virus can potentially cross the placenta and infect the developing fetus, leading to congenital CMV. While many infected pregnant women may be asymptomatic or experience only mild symptoms, some may develop a mononucleosis-like illness with fever, fatigue, and swollen lymph nodes.

- **Immunocompromised Individuals:**

  Individuals with weakened immune systems, such as organ transplant recipients, cancer patients undergoing chemotherapy or radiation therapy, and those living with

HIV/AIDS, are at an increased risk of severe CMV infections. Symptoms can vary depending on the organ system affected; however, they may include pneumonia, gastrointestinal disease, retinitis (potentially leading to vision loss), hepatitis, and encephalitis.

- **Older Adults:**
  In older adults, particularly those with underlying medical conditions or weakened immune systems, CMV infection can cause more severe symptoms and complications, such as pneumonia, gastroenteritis, and neurological problems. Reactivation of a latent CMV infection in this population can also contribute to frailty and exacerbate existing health issues.

By understanding the diverse presentation of CMV symptoms across different demographic groups, healthcare professionals can better recognize potential infections, initiate appropriate diagnostic testing, and provide prompt treatment and management strategies tailored to the individual's age, immune status, and overall health.

When to Seek Medical Attention

While cytomegalovirus (CMV) infections are often asymptomatic or cause only mild, flu-like symptoms in healthy individuals, there are certain situations where seeking prompt medical attention is crucial. Recognizing these circumstances can help prevent complications and ensure appropriate infection management, especially for high-risk groups.

- **Prolonged or Severe Symptoms:** Suppose you experience symptoms such as high fever, extreme fatigue, severe headaches, persistent muscle aches, and swollen lymph nodes that last more than a week or two. In that case, you should consult a healthcare provider. These symptoms could indicate a more severe CMV infection or complications, particularly in individuals with weakened immune systems.

- **Symptoms in Newborns and Infants:**
  Any signs of illness in newborns or infants, such as poor feeding, jaundice, rash, or neurological abnormalities, should prompt immediate medical evaluation. Congenital CMV can have severe consequences for the developing child, and early diagnosis and treatment are essential to minimize the potential impact.

- **Pregnancy:**
  If you are pregnant and suspect that you may have contracted CMV, it is crucial to seek medical attention promptly. Your healthcare provider can order appropriate tests to confirm the infection and provide guidance on managing the potential risks to your unborn child, including monitoring for congenital CMV and discussing available treatment options.

- **Immunocompromised Individuals:**
  Individuals with weakened immune systems, such as organ transplant recipients, cancer patients undergoing chemotherapy or

radiation therapy, and those living with HIV/AIDS, should seek medical attention at the earliest signs of CMV-related symptoms. These may include fever, cough, shortness of breath, vision problems, or neurological symptoms. CMV can cause severe complications in immunocompromised individuals.

- **Persistent or Worsening Symptoms After Treatment:**
Suppose you have been diagnosed with CMV and have started treatment, but your symptoms persist or worsen despite appropriate management. In that case, it is essential to consult your healthcare provider. This could indicate a need for adjustments in treatment or further evaluation for potential complications.

- **Concerns or Uncertainty:**
Even if symptoms seem mild or nonspecific, it is always better to consult a healthcare professional if you have concerns or uncertainties about the possibility of a CMV

infection. They can provide guidance, order appropriate tests, and address any questions or concerns you may have regarding the infection.

By seeking medical attention promptly in these situations, individuals can receive timely diagnosis, appropriate treatment, and guidance on managing the potential risks and complications associated with CMV infection. Early intervention and proper management are crucial for protecting the health and well-being of those affected, especially vulnerable populations such as newborns, pregnant women, and individuals with weakened immune systems.

Chapter 4

DIAGNOSIS AND TESTING

Laboratory Tests for CMV

Accurate cytomegalovirus (CMV) infection diagnosis is essential for effective management and treatment, especially in high-risk populations. Several laboratory tests are available to detect the presence of the virus, measure the body's immune response, and determine the stage and severity of the infection.

- **Viral Culture:**

  Viral culture is a traditional diagnostic method that involves growing the virus from a sample of bodily fluids, such as blood, urine, or respiratory secretions. While this method is highly specific, it is time-consuming and may take several weeks to obtain results. Viral culture is typically used to diagnose congenital CMV in newborns or monitor the progression of CMV infection in immunocompromised individuals.

- **Polymerase Chain Reaction (PCR) Testing:**

  PCR testing is a highly sensitive and specific molecular diagnostic technique that can detect the presence of CMV DNA or RNA in various bodily fluids, including blood, urine, and cerebrospinal fluid (CSF). This test is particularly useful for diagnosing active CMV infections, monitoring viral load, and assessing the effectiveness of antiviral treatment.

- **Serology Testing:**

  Serology tests, such as enzyme-linked immunosorbent assays (ELISA) or immunofluorescence assays, detect the presence of antibodies against CMV in the patient's blood. These tests can help determine if an individual has been previously exposed to the virus and can aid in diagnosing primary or reactivated CMV infections.

- **Antigenemia Assay:**
The antigenemia assay is a specialized test that detects the presence of CMV antigens in the patient's blood. This test is commonly used to monitor the viral load and assess the risk of CMV disease in immunocompromised patients, such as organ transplant recipients or individuals receiving chemotherapy.

- **Histopathology and Immunohistochemistry:**
In some cases, tissue biopsies may be performed, and the samples are examined under a microscope for the presence of characteristic cytomegalic cells or viral antigens. Histopathological and immunohistochemical analyses can provide valuable information about the involvement of specific organs or tissues in the CMV infection.

The choice of diagnostic test depends on various factors, including the patient's age, immune status, clinical presentation, and the suspected stage of the infection. In many cases, a combination of tests may be used to understand the CMV infection and guide appropriate treatment decisions comprehensively.

Accurate diagnosis is crucial for initiating prompt and effective management strategies, protecting high-risk individuals, and preventing potential complications associated with CMV infection.

Imaging and Other Diagnostic Tools

While laboratory tests are the primary diagnostic tools for detecting and monitoring cytomegalovirus (CMV) infections, various imaging techniques and other diagnostic methods can provide valuable information about the virus's extent and impact on different organ systems.

- **Imaging Techniques:**
    a. ***Computed Tomography (CT) Scans:*** CT scans can detect CMV-related organ involvement, such as pneumonia, hepatitis, or central

nervous system (CNS) abnormalities. These detailed images can help identify the location and severity of the infection.

b. ***Magnetic Resonance Imaging (MRI):*** MRI is particularly valuable in evaluating CMV-related neurological complications, such as encephalitis or brain lesions. It can provide high-resolution images of the brain and spinal cord, aiding in diagnosing and monitoring CMV-related neurological manifestations.

c. ***Ultrasonography:*** Prenatal ultrasonography can play a crucial role in detecting signs of congenital CMV infection in utero, such as fetal growth restriction, brain calcifications, or abnormalities in organ development.

d. ***Fundoscopic Examination:*** For individuals at risk of CMV-related retinitis, a fundoscopic examination can help identify and monitor any abnormalities or lesions in the retina caused by the virus.

- **Ophthalmological Evaluation:** Comprehensive ophthalmological evaluations, including visual acuity testing, slit-lamp examination, and fundoscopy, are essential for diagnosing and monitoring CMV-related eye diseases, such as retinitis or optic neuritis. These evaluations can help detect early signs of vision impairment and guide appropriate treatment.

- **Auditory Testing:** Hearing assessments, including auditory brainstem response (ABR) testing and otoacoustic emissions (OAE) testing, are crucial for diagnosing and monitoring sensorineural hearing loss associated with congenital CMV infections. Early detection and intervention are vital for minimizing the impact on speech and language development in affected infants.

- **Developmental and Neurological Assessments:**

  For infants and children with congenital CMV or CMV-related neurological complications, regular developmental and neurological assessments are essential. These evaluations can help identify and track any delays or impairments in cognitive, motor, or sensory functions, allowing for early intervention and support strategies.

- **Invasive Procedures:**

  In certain cases, invasive diagnostic procedures, such as tissue biopsies or lumbar punctures, may be necessary to obtain samples for laboratory testing or to evaluate the involvement of specific organs or tissues in the CMV infection.

The integration of imaging techniques, specialized evaluations, and other diagnostic tools with laboratory testing provides a comprehensive approach to diagnosing and monitoring CMV infections. This multidisciplinary approach is particularly important in high-risk populations, such as newborns, pregnant women, and immunocompromised individuals, where early detection and accurate assessment of the infection's impact are crucial for optimal management and prevention of potential complications.

Interpreting Test Results

Interpreting the results of cytomegalovirus (CMV) diagnostic tests requires careful consideration of various factors, as the interpretation can vary depending on the patient's age, immune status, and clinical presentation. Understanding the nuances of test result interpretation is crucial for accurate diagnosis, appropriate treatment decisions, and effective management of CMV infections.

- **Viral Culture and PCR Testing:**
  a. A positive viral culture or PCR test confirms the presence of active CMV infection.
  b. In immunocompetent individuals, a positive result may indicate a primary infection or reactivation of a latent infection.

   c. A positive result in immunocompromised patients can signify an active and potentially severe CMV infection requiring prompt treatment.

   d. Quantitative PCR tests can provide information about viral load, which can help assess the severity of the infection and monitor treatment response.

- **Serology Testing:**
  a. CMV-specific immunoglobulin M (IgM) antibodies suggest a recent or primary CMV infection.
  b. CMV-specific immunoglobulin G (IgG) antibodies indicate a past infection or exposure to the virus.
  c. In immunocompetent individuals, IgG antibodies alone may indicate a latent or reactivated infection.
  d. In immunocompromised patients, the absence of IgG antibodies can indicate a higher risk of severe CMV disease.

- **Antigenemia Assay:**
    a. This test is primarily used to monitor CMV infection in immunocompromised patients, such as organ transplant recipients or individuals receiving chemotherapy.
    b. A high antigenemia level is associated with an increased risk of CMV disease and may warrant preemptive or therapeutic antiviral treatment.
    c. Serial antigenemia testing can help evaluate the effectiveness of antiviral therapy and guide treatment decisions.

- **Histopathology and Immunohistochemistry:**
    a. The presence of characteristic cytomegalic cells or viral antigens in tissue samples can confirm CMV involvement in specific organs or tissues.
    b. Combined with clinical presentation, these findings can help diagnose CMV-related diseases, such as pneumonitis, hepatitis, or encephalitis.

When interpreting CMV test results, it is essential to consider the patient's overall clinical picture, including symptoms, immune status, and potential risk factors. Additionally, healthcare professionals should be aware of the limitations and potential for false-positive or false-negative results with certain tests and the possibility of cross-reactivity with other viruses.

In many cases, a combination of different diagnostic tests may be necessary to understand the CMV infection and make informed treatment decisions comprehensively. Close collaboration between healthcare providers, laboratory professionals, and infectious disease specialists is vital for accurate test interpretation and optimal management of CMV infections, particularly in high-risk populations.

Chapter 5

TREATMENT STRATEGIES

Antiviral Medications

Antiviral medications play a crucial role in treating and managing cytomegalovirus (CMV) infections, particularly in high-risk populations such as individuals with weakened immune systems, newborns with congenital CMV, and pregnant women with primary CMV infections during pregnancy. The following antiviral drugs are commonly used in the treatment of CMV infections:

- **Ganciclovir:**

  Ganciclovir is a nucleoside analog antiviral medication widely used as the primary treatment for CMV infections. It works by inhibiting the viral DNA polymerase, thereby preventing the virus's replication. Ganciclovir can be administered intravenously or orally (as the prodrug valganciclovir).

- **Valganciclovir:**
Valganciclovir is an oral prodrug that is metabolized into ganciclovir in the body. It provides a convenient oral treatment option for certain CMV infections and is commonly used for the treatment and prevention of CMV disease in solid organ and bone marrow transplant recipients.

- **Foscarnet:**
Foscarnet is a pyrophosphate analog antiviral medication that inhibits the viral DNA polymerase and reverses transcriptase, preventing viral replication. It is primarily used as a second-line treatment option for CMV infections in cases where resistance to ganciclovir or valganciclovir has developed or when these drugs are contraindicated due to adverse effects or toxicity concerns.

- **Cidofovir:**

  Cidofovir is a nucleotide analogue antiviral medication that inhibits the viral DNA polymerase, thereby preventing viral DNA synthesis and replication. It is primarily used as a third-line treatment option for CMV retinitis in patients with AIDS or for other resistant or refractory CMV infections.

- **Letermovir:**

  Letermovir is a newer antiviral medication that inhibits the viral terminase complex, which is essential for viral DNA packaging and replication. It is approved for the prophylaxis (prevention) of CMV infection and disease in adult CMV-seropositive recipients of an allogeneic hematopoietic stem cell transplant.

The choice of antiviral medication, dosage, and duration of treatment depends on various factors, including the patient's age, immune status, organ involvement, and the severity of the CMV infection. In some cases, a combination of antiviral drugs may enhance treatment efficacy or overcome potential drug resistance.

It is important to note that antiviral medications can have significant side effects and toxicities, particularly with prolonged use or in immunocompromised patients. Close monitoring by healthcare professionals is essential to ensure the safe and effective use of these medications and manage any adverse effects that may arise.

Antiviral therapy, coupled with appropriate supportive care and management of underlying conditions, is vital in controlling CMV infections, reducing the risk of severe complications, and improving clinical outcomes, especially in high-risk populations.

Supportive Care Options

While antiviral medications are the cornerstone of treatment for cytomegalovirus (CMV) infections, supportive care measures play a crucial role in managing patients' symptoms, complications, and overall well-being, particularly those in high-risk groups or with severe infections.

- **Hydration and Nutritional Support:** CMV infections can cause significant fatigue, loss of appetite, and gastrointestinal disturbances, leading to dehydration and malnutrition. Ensuring adequate hydration through intravenous fluids or oral rehydration solutions and providing nutritional support through enteral or parenteral feeding may be necessary in severe cases to maintain overall health and support the body's ability to fight the infection.

- **Management of Organ-Specific Complications:** Various supportive care measures may be required, depending on the organ systems affected by the CMV infection. For example, in cases of CMV pneumonia, oxygen therapy or mechanical ventilation may be necessary to support respiratory function. In cases of CMV retinitis, ophthalmological interventions, such as intravitreal injections of antivirals or vitrectomy, may be required to preserve vision.

- **Pain Management:** CMV infections can cause significant discomfort and pain, particularly in cases of organ involvement or complications. Appropriate pain management strategies, including the use of analgesics and other pain-relieving interventions, can improve the patient's quality of life and facilitate recovery.

- **Infection Control Measures:** Strict adherence to infection control protocols is crucial to preventing the spread of CMV, especially in healthcare settings and among high-risk populations. Measures such as proper hand hygiene, the use of personal protective equipment (PPE), and isolation precautions may be necessary to minimize the risk of transmission.

- **Rehabilitation and Supportive Therapies:** For patients who experience long-term complications or disabilities as a result of CMV infection, such as hearing loss, vision impairment, or developmental delays, rehabilitation, and supportive therapies can play a vital role in improving quality of life and promoting functional recovery. These may include speech and language therapy, physical therapy, occupational therapy, and educational interventions.

- **Psychosocial Support:** The impact of CMV infections, particularly in cases of congenital CMV or severe complications, can be emotionally and psychologically overwhelming for patients and their families. Providing access to counseling, support groups, and mental health services can help individuals cope with the challenges and stresses of the condition.

Supportive care measures should be tailored to the individual patient's needs and integrated into a comprehensive treatment plan that addresses the underlying CMV infection, potential complications, and associated challenges. By combining antiviral therapy with appropriate supportive care strategies, healthcare professionals can optimize clinical outcomes, minimize the impact of the infection, and improve the overall well-being of patients affected by CMV.

Emerging Therapies

While currently available antiviral medications and supportive care measures have significantly improved cytomegalovirus (CMV) infection management, ongoing research efforts are focused on developing new and innovative therapies to address the persistent virus's challenges further. Several promising emerging therapies are currently under investigation, offering potential advancements in treating and preventing CMV-related diseases.

- **Novel Antiviral Agents:**
  Researchers are actively exploring new antiviral compounds with different mechanisms of action to combat CMV infections, particularly in cases of drug resistance or treatment failure with existing antivirals. Some of the novel antiviral agents under investigation include:

  a. **Maribavir:** A benzimidazole antiviral that inhibits the viral protein kinase UL97, thereby disrupting viral replication. Maribavir has shown promise in treating drug-resistant CMV infections and is currently undergoing clinical trials.

b. **Brincidofovir:** A lipid-conjugated nucleotide analogue that inhibits viral DNA synthesis. Brincidofovir has demonstrated potential in treating CMV infections in hematopoietic stem cell transplant recipients and is being evaluated for various indications, including the treatment of adenovirus infections.

- **Immunotherapeutic Approaches:**
Harnessing the immune system's power to combat CMV infections is an area of active research. Immunotherapeutic strategies under investigation include:

a. **CMV-specific T-cell therapies:** These involve the isolation, expansion, and infusion of CMV-specific T-cells from the patient or a donor to enhance the immune response against the virus. Clinical trials have shown promising results in preventing and treating CMV infections in immunocompromised patients.

b. **Monoclonal antibodies:** Monoclonal antibodies targeting specific CMV proteins or antigens are being explored as potential immunotherapeutic agents. These antibodies could neutralize the virus, block entry into host cells, or enhance the immune response against CMV.

- **Gene Therapy and Genetic Approaches:** Emerging genetic technologies, such as gene editing and RNA interference (RNAi), are being explored as potential strategies for targeting and disrupting CMV infections at the molecular level. These approaches aim to manipulate cellular pathways or viral genes to inhibit viral replication or enhance the host's antiviral defenses.

While many of these emerging therapies are still in the early stages of development and clinical testing, they represent promising avenues for improving the management and prevention of CMV infections, particularly in high-risk populations and cases where current treatment options are limited or ineffective. Continued research, collaboration, and investment in these innovative approaches are crucial for advancing our understanding and ability to combat this persistent viral threat.

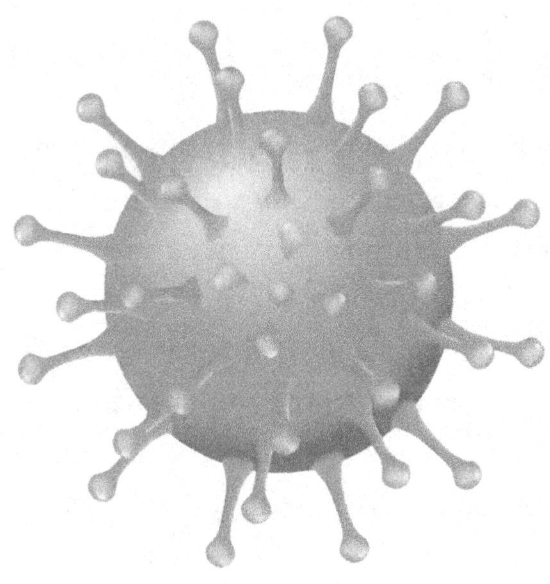

Chapter 6

LIVING WITH CMV

Daily Management of CMV

For individuals living with cytomegalovirus (CMV) infections, particularly those in high-risk groups or experiencing chronic or recurrent symptoms, implementing effective daily management strategies is crucial for maintaining overall health, reducing the risk of complications, and improving quality of life. While the specific management approach may vary depending on the individual's age, immune status, and severity of the infection, several vital aspects should be considered.

- **Adhering to Treatment Regimens:** Strict adherence to prescribed antiviral medication regimens is essential for successfully managing CMV infections. Patients should take their medications as directed, without skipping doses or altering the dosage without consulting their healthcare provider. Maintaining consistent treatment can help control viral replication, reduce the risk of complications, and prevent the development of drug resistance.

- **Monitoring and Reporting Symptoms:** Individuals living with CMV infections should be vigilant about monitoring their symptoms and promptly reporting any changes or ncw concerns to their healthcare team. Regular check-ups and follow-up appointments can help healthcare providers assess the effectiveness of treatment, adjust medication dosages if needed, and promptly address any complications or side effects.

- **Practicing Good Hygiene:** Implementing good hygiene practices can help prevent the spread of CMV and reduce the risk of reinfection or reactivation. This includes frequent handwashing, covering coughs and sneezes, avoiding sharing personal items like utensils or drinking containers and practicing safe handling of bodily fluids.

- **Managing Stress and Fatigue:** CMV infections can often cause significant fatigue and emotional stress, particularly in cases of chronic or severe illness. Incorporating stress management techniques, such as meditation, yoga, or counseling, and prioritizing rest and self-care can help individuals cope with the physical and emotional demands of living with CMV.

- **Maintaining a Balanced Diet:** A nutritious and balanced diet can support overall health and provide the body with the resources to fight infections effectively. Individuals with CMV should consult with a dietitian or healthcare provider to develop a meal plan that meets their nutritional needs and accommodates dietary restrictions or intolerances.

- **Staying Active:** As tolerated and recommended by healthcare providers, regular physical activity can help maintain overall fitness, reduce stress, and promote a sense of well-being. Low-impact exercises like walking, swimming, or light yoga can benefit individuals living with CMV.

- **Building a Support System:** Living with CMV can be challenging, both physically and emotionally. Building a strong support system through family, friends, support groups, or counseling services can provide a valuable source of encouragement, understanding, and practical assistance.

By integrating these daily management strategies into their routine, individuals living with CMV can actively participate in their care and take proactive steps to minimize the impact of the infection on their overall well-being. Close collaboration with healthcare professionals and open communication about concerns or challenges are essential for tailoring the management approach to each individual's unique needs and circumstances.

Long-Term Health Considerations

While cytomegalovirus (CMV) infections are often self-limiting and may resolve without significant complications in healthy individuals, certain populations, including those with weakened immune systems, newborns with congenital CMV, and individuals with severe or recurrent infections, may face long-term health considerations that require careful monitoring and management.

- **Chronic Organ Damage:**
  In some cases, CMV infections can lead to chronic or progressive damage to various organs, such as the lungs, liver, gastrointestinal tract, or eyes. Regular monitoring and follow-up with healthcare professionals are essential to assess organ function, detect any ongoing or residual damage, and implement appropriate interventions or treatments to minimize further deterioration.

- **Neurological Complications:**
CMV infections, particularly congenital CMV, can have long-term neurological implications, including developmental delays, intellectual disabilities, seizures, and hearing or vision impairments. Individuals affected by these complications may require ongoing specialized care, such as speech and language therapy, occupational therapy, or educational support services, to address their specific needs and promote optimal development and quality of life.

- **Secondary Infections:**
CMV infections can weaken the immune system, increasing the risk of secondary bacterial, fungal, or viral infections. Individuals with chronic or recurrent CMV infections may need regular monitoring for opportunistic infections and appropriate prophylactic or therapeutic interventions to prevent or manage these complications.

- **Immune System Monitoring:**
  In immunocompromised individuals, such as organ transplant recipients or those with HIV/AIDS, regular monitoring of the immune system function is crucial. This may involve periodic tests to assess immune cell counts, antibody levels, overall immune competence, and adjustments to immunosuppressive therapies or treatment regimens as needed.

- **Emotional and Psychological Support:**
  Living with the long-term effects of CMV infections, particularly in cases of congenital CMV or severe complications, can take an emotional and psychological toll on individuals and their families. Access to mental health services, counseling, and support groups can be invaluable in coping with the challenges, managing stress and anxiety, and promoting overall well-being.

- **Lifestyle Modifications:**
  Depending on the severity and complications of the CMV infection, individuals may need to make long-term lifestyle adjustments to

accommodate their health needs. This could include modifying dietary habits, implementing stress management techniques, engaging in appropriate physical activities, or making environmental modifications to improve accessibility or reduce exposure to potential sources of infection.

Effective long-term management of CMV infections requires a multidisciplinary approach involving healthcare professionals from various specialties, such as infectious disease specialists, neurologists, ophthalmologists, and mental health professionals.

Lifestyle Adjustments and Coping Strategies

Living with cytomegalovirus (CMV) infections, particularly for those in high-risk groups or experiencing chronic or recurrent symptoms, may require lifestyle adjustments and effective coping strategies to manage the physical, emotional, and practical challenges associated with the condition.

- **Prioritizing Rest and Energy Conservation:** CMV infections can cause significant fatigue and weakness, making it essential to prioritize rest and energy conservation. Individuals may need to adjust their daily routines, reduce their workload, or delegate tasks to manage their energy levels more effectively. Incorporating regular rest periods, napping, or engaging in relaxation techniques like meditation or deep breathing exercises can help combat fatigue and promote overall well-being.

- **Adapting Dietary Habits:** Maintaining a balanced and nutritious diet is crucial for supporting overall health and the body's ability to fight infections. Individuals with CMV may need to modify their dietary habits based on their specific needs and any associated complications or side effects of treatment. Working with a registered dietitian or nutritionist can help develop an individualized meal plan that addresses specific nutritional requirements, food intolerances, or dietary restrictions.

- **Practicing Good Hygiene and Infection Control:** Adhering to strict hygiene practices and infection control measures is essential for preventing the spread of CMV and reducing the risk of reinfection or reactivation. This includes frequent handwashing, avoiding sharing personal items, practicing safe handling of bodily fluids, and following any additional precautions recommended by healthcare professionals, especially in healthcare settings or when interacting with high-risk individuals.

- **Stress Management and Emotional Support:** Living with CMV can be emotionally and psychologically challenging, particularly when dealing with chronic symptoms, complications, or the impact on daily life. Incorporating stress management techniques, such as mindfulness practices, counseling, or joining support groups, can help individuals cope with the emotional demands of the condition and foster a sense of connection and understanding.

- **Engaging in Physical Activity:** As tolerated and recommended by healthcare providers, regular, low-impact physical activity can help maintain overall fitness, reduce stress, and promote a sense of well-being. Activities like walking, swimming, or gentle yoga can benefit individuals living with CMV, provided they are tailored to individual capabilities and limitations.

- **Building a Support Network:** Developing a strong support network can be invaluable for individuals living with CMV. This network may include family members, friends, support groups, or online communities that can offer practical assistance, emotional support, and a sense of shared understanding.

- **Staying Informed and Advocating for Yourself:** Educating oneself about CMV, its potential complications, and available treatments can empower individuals to make informed decisions about their care and effectively advocate for their needs. Maintaining open communication with healthcare professionals, asking questions, and actively participating in treatment decisions can improve overall outcomes and quality of life.

Chapter 7

SPECIAL POPULATIONS

CMV in Pregnancy

Cytomegalovirus (CMV) infection during pregnancy is a significant concern due to the potential risk of transmitting the virus to the developing fetus, a condition known as congenital CMV. Congenital CMV can lead to severe congenital disabilities and long-term disabilities, making it crucial for pregnant women and their healthcare providers to be aware of the risks, preventive measures, and appropriate management strategies.

- **Risks and Consequences:**
  - Primary CMV infection during pregnancy poses the highest risk of

congenital transmission, with rates ranging from 30% to 40%.

- Congenital CMV can result in a range of congenital disabilities, including hearing loss, vision impairment, intellectual disabilities, seizures, and developmental delays.
- The severity of the effects on the fetus depends on the timing of the infection during pregnancy, with infections occurring earlier in gestation generally associated with more severe outcomes.

- **Preventive Measures:**
  - Practicing good hygiene, such as frequent handwashing and avoiding sharing utensils or cups, can reduce the risk of contracting CMV during pregnancy.
  - Avoiding close contact with young children, who are a common source of CMV transmission, can also help prevent infection.

- Healthcare workers should follow strict infection control protocols to minimize occupational exposure to CMV.

- **Screening and Diagnosis:**
  - Routine screening for CMV during pregnancy is not universally recommended, but it may be considered for women with specific risk factors or in areas with high CMV prevalence.
  - If a primary CMV infection is suspected during pregnancy, diagnostic tests such as serology (testing for CMV-specific antibodies) or PCR (detecting viral DNA) can be performed.
  - Prenatal ultrasound and fetal MRI may be used to assess for potential congenital abnormalities or signs of fetal infection.

- **Management and Treatment:**
  - If a primary CMV infection is confirmed during pregnancy, close

monitoring of the fetus, including regular ultrasounds and fetal testing, is recommended.

- Antiviral medications, such as valganciclovir or ganciclovir, may be considered for pregnant women with primary CMV infections, particularly in cases of fetal involvement or severe maternal illness.

- Delivery management, including the potential need for a cesarean section, will depend on the severity of the infection and the presence of fetal complications.

- **Postpartum Care:**
  - Newborns with congenital CMV may require specialized care, including hearing and vision assessments, developmental evaluations, and potential antiviral treatment.
  - Long-term follow-up and supportive services, such as early intervention programs and therapies, may be

necessary for infants affected by congenital CMV.

Effective prevention, early detection, and appropriate management of CMV during pregnancy are crucial to minimizing the risk of congenital transmission and the potential for severe congenital disabilities and long-term disabilities. Close collaboration between pregnant women, obstetricians, and healthcare teams is essential to ensuring the best possible outcomes for both mother and child.

CMV in Immunocompromised Individuals

Individuals with compromised immune systems, such as organ transplant recipients, cancer patients undergoing chemotherapy or radiation therapy, and those living with HIV/AIDS, are at a significantly higher risk of developing severe and life-threatening complications from cytomegalovirus (CMV) infections. In these populations, CMV can reactivate from a latent state or cause a primary infection, leading to potentially devastating outcomes.

- **Risks and Consequences:**
  - CMV is a leading cause of viral infections and disease in immunocompromised individuals, contributing to increased morbidity and mortality rates.
  - In solid organ transplant recipients, CMV can cause organ rejection, graft failure, and various end-organ diseases, such as pneumonia, hepatitis, and gastrointestinal disease.
  - In hematopoietic stem cell transplant (HSCT) recipients, CMV can lead to severe complications, including pneumonia, enteritis, retinitis, and an increased risk of graft-versus-host disease (GVHD).
  - In individuals with HIV/AIDS, CMV can cause retinitis, leading to vision loss, as well as other severe systemic infections affecting various organs.

- **Preventive Strategies:**
  - Screening for CMV status (serological testing) before transplantation or immunosuppressive therapy is crucial for risk stratification and guiding preventive strategies.
  - Antiviral prophylaxis with medications like valganciclovir or ganciclovir may be administered to high-risk patients to prevent CMV reactivation or disease.
  - Strict infection control measures, such as hand hygiene, isolation precautions, and proper bodily fluid handling, are essential to prevent the transmission of CMV in healthcare settings.

- **Monitoring and Diagnosis:**
  - Regular CMV reactivation or disease monitoring is critical for immunocompromised individuals, typically through viral load testing (PCR) or antigenemia assays.
  - Early detection of CMV infection or reactivation is crucial for prompt

initiation of treatment and prevention of end-organ disease.

- Diagnostic procedures, such as biopsies or imaging studies, may be required to confirm CMV involvement in specific organs or tissues.

- **Treatment and Management:**
  - Antiviral medications, such as ganciclovir, valganciclovir, foscarnet, or cidofovir, are the mainstay of treatment for CMV infections in immunocompromised individuals.
  - The choice of antiviral agent, dosage, and treatment duration depends on the severity of the infection, the patient's immune status, and the presence of drug resistance.
  - Supportive care, such as hydration, nutritional support, and management of organ-specific complications, is essential for optimal outcomes.
  - In severe or refractory cases, novel antiviral agents, immunotherapies, or

a combination of treatment modalities may be considered.

Effective prevention, early detection, and prompt treatment of CMV infections in immunocompromised individuals are crucial to minimize the risk of severe complications and improve overall outcomes. Close collaboration between infectious disease specialists, transplant teams, oncologists, and other healthcare professionals is essential for optimal management and care of these high-risk patients.

Pediatric CMV

Cytomegalovirus (CMV) infections in children can have significant implications, particularly in the case of congenital CMV, which occurs when the virus is transmitted from an infected mother to her unborn child during pregnancy. Pediatric CMV also poses risks for children with weakened immune systems or those undergoing organ transplantation.

- **Congenital CMV:**
  - Congenital CMV is one of the most common congenital infections,

affecting approximately 1 in 200 newborns worldwide.

- It can lead to a range of congenital disabilities and long-term disabilities, including hearing loss, vision impairment, intellectual disabilities, seizures, and developmental delays.
- The severity of the effects on the fetus depends on the timing of the infection during pregnancy, with infections occurring earlier in gestation generally associated with more severe outcomes.
- Infants with symptomatic congenital CMV may exhibit features such as petechial rashes, jaundice, hepatosplenomegaly (enlarged liver and spleen), and neurological abnormalities.

- **Acquired CMV in Children:**
  - Most healthy children who acquire CMV after birth experience no symptoms or only mild, flu-like symptoms.

- However, in children with weakened immune systems, such as those undergoing chemotherapy or organ transplantation, CMV can cause severe complications, including pneumonia, hepatitis, and gastrointestinal disease.

- **Diagnosis and Screening:**
  - Diagnostic tests for congenital CMV may include PCR testing of saliva, urine, or blood samples from the newborn and prenatal testing during pregnancy (serology, PCR, or ultrasound).
  - Screening for congenital CMV is not universally recommended, but it may be considered in high-risk populations or areas with high CMV prevalence.
  - In children with acquired CMV infections, diagnostic tests may include serological testing (for antibodies) or PCR testing for viral DNA.

- **Treatment and Management:**
  - Antiviral medications, such as ganciclovir or valganciclovir, may be prescribed for infants with symptomatic congenital CMV or severe acquired CMV infections in immunocompromised children.
  - Supportive care, such as hearing and vision assessments, developmental evaluations, and early intervention therapies (e.g., speech, occupational, physical), are crucial for infants with congenital CMV.
  - Long-term follow-up and monitoring for potential late-onset complications, such as hearing loss or developmental delays, are essential for children with congenital CMV.

Close collaboration between pediatricians, obstetricians, infectious disease specialists, and other healthcare professionals is essential for ensuring the best possible outcomes for affected children and their families.

Chapter 8

ADVANCES IN RESEARCH

Recent Scientific Discoveries

The field of cytomegalovirus (CMV) research has witnessed significant advancements in recent years, driven by the ongoing pursuit of understanding this complex virus and developing more effective prevention, diagnosis, and treatment strategies. These scientific discoveries have shed light on CMV biology, pathogenesis, and host-virus interactions, paving the way for potential breakthroughs in combating this persistent viral threat.

- **Viral Entry and Host Cell Interactions:** Researchers have made strides in unraveling the intricate mechanisms by which CMV enters and manipulates host cells. These discoveries have revealed the viral entry receptors, the role of viral proteins in hijacking cellular pathways, and the strategies CMV employs to evade the host's immune defenses. This knowledge has opened avenues for exploring novel therapeutic targets and developing interventions that can disrupt the viral life cycle at various stages.

- **Immune Response and Viral Evasion Tactics:** Significant progress has been made in understanding the complex interplay between CMV and the host's immune system. Scientists have identified key viral proteins and mechanisms that enable CMV to evade immune recognition and suppress immune responses. These discoveries have provided insights into potential strategies for enhancing immune surveillance and developing immunotherapeutic approaches against CMV infections.

- **Genomics and Molecular Epidemiology:** Advances in genomic technologies have enabled researchers to study the genetic diversity and evolution of CMV strains. By sequencing and analyzing the genomes of different CMV isolates, scientists have gained valuable insights into the virus's genetic variability, potential virulence factors, and the emergence of drug-resistance mutations. This knowledge can inform the development of more effective diagnostic tools, targeted therapies, and potential vaccine candidates.

- **Antiviral Drug Development:** The search for novel antiviral agents against CMV has intensified, driven by the need to address drug resistance and improve therapeutic options for high-risk populations. Researchers have explored new classes of compounds with different mechanisms of action, such as nucleoside analogs, protease inhibitors, and terminase inhibitors. Some of these investigational drugs have shown promising results in preclinical and clinical studies, offering potential alternatives to existing antiviral therapies.

- **Vaccine Development Efforts:** The quest for an effective CMV vaccine has been a long-standing endeavor in viral immunology. Researchers have explored various vaccine platforms, including live-attenuated, subunit, and vectored vaccines, intending to induce robust and long-lasting immune responses against CMV. While no licensed CMV vaccine is currently available, several vaccine candidates have shown promising results in clinical trials, reigniting hopes for a preventive solution against this widespread viral infection.

These recent scientific discoveries have deepened our understanding of CMV and opened up new avenues for potential interventions and therapeutic strategies. Collaborative efforts among researchers, healthcare professionals, and regulatory agencies will be crucial in translating these scientific advancements into tangible benefits for individuals at risk of or affected by CMV infections.

Vaccine Development

The development of an effective and safe vaccine against cytomegalovirus (CMV) has been a long-standing goal in viral immunology and vaccine research. While no licensed CMV vaccine is currently available, significant progress has been made in recent years, with several promising vaccine candidates advancing through various stages of clinical development.

- **Challenges in CMV Vaccine Development:**
  - CMV is a complex virus with a large genome, making it challenging to identify and target the most effective antigens for inducing protective immunity.
  - The virus can evade and modulate the host's immune system through various mechanisms, complicating the development of a vaccine that can elicit a robust and long-lasting immune response.

- Diverse populations, including newborns, pregnant women, and immunocompromised individuals, may require different vaccine strategies tailored to their needs and immune responses.

- **Vaccine Platforms and Approaches:**
  - ***Live-attenuated vaccines:*** These vaccines use a weakened or attenuated form of the CMV virus to stimulate an immune response. While potentially effective, safety concerns have hindered their development for use in certain populations, such as pregnant women and immunocompromised individuals.
  - ***Subunit vaccines:*** These vaccines contain specific CMV proteins or protein complexes designed to elicit a targeted immune response against the virus. Researchers have explored various CMV antigens, including glycoprotein B (gB) and the pentameric

complex (PC), as potential vaccine candidates.

- ○ ***Vectored vaccines:*** These vaccines use harmless viruses or bacteria as vectors to deliver CMV antigens and stimulate an immune response. Viral vectors, such as modified vaccinia or adenoviruses, have been explored as potential delivery platforms for CMV vaccines.

- ○ ***Prime-boost strategies:*** Researchers are investigating the use of different vaccine platforms in a prime-boost approach, where an initial vaccine primes the immune system, and a subsequent booster vaccine further enhances and strengthens the immune response against CMV.

- **Clinical Trials and Promising Candidates:**

    - ○ Several CMV vaccine candidates have shown promising results in preclinical studies and early-stage clinical trials, demonstrating their ability to induce robust immune responses and potential efficacy in preventing CMV infection or disease.

- o Notable candidates include the gB/MF59 subunit vaccine, the V160 bivalent vaccine (containing gB and the PC), and the mRNA-based vaccine approach, which utilizes messenger RNA technology to deliver CMV antigens.
- o Ongoing clinical trials are evaluating the safety, immunogenicity, and potential efficacy of these vaccine candidates in various target populations, including healthy adults, adolescents, pregnant women, and transplant recipients.

While significant challenges remain, the progress in CMV vaccine development represents a promising step towards potentially reducing the global burden of CMV infections and protecting vulnerable populations from the devastating consequences of this persistent viral threat.

The Future of CMV Treatment

The future of cytomegalovirus (CMV) treatment holds promising prospects as ongoing research and scientific advancements shed light on new and innovative approaches to combat this persistent viral threat. While current antiviral medications and supportive care measures have significantly improved the management of CMV infections, the limitations of existing therapies and the emergence of drug resistance highlight the need for novel treatment strategies.

Novel Antiviral Agents:

Researchers are actively exploring new classes of antiviral compounds with unique mechanisms of action to overcome current therapies' limitations and address the drug resistance challenge. Some promising investigational agents include:

- **Letermovir:** A recently approved antiviral that inhibits the viral terminase complex, preventing viral DNA packaging and replication. Letermovir is approved for prophylaxis of CMV infection in certain transplant recipients.

- **Maribavir:** A benzimidazole antiviral that inhibits viral protein kinase UL97, disrupting viral replication. Maribavir has shown potential for treating drug-resistant CMV infections.

- **Brincidofovir:** A lipid-conjugated nucleotide analogue that inhibits viral DNA synthesis, currently under investigation for various indications, including treating CMV infections.

Immunotherapeutic Approaches:

Harnessing the immune system to fight CMV infections is an active area of research. Immunotherapeutic strategies under investigation include:

- **CMV-specific T-cell therapies:** These involve the isolation, expansion, and infusion of CMV-specific T-cells from the patient or a donor to enhance the immune response against the virus.

- **Monoclonal antibodies:** Monoclonal antibodies targeting specific CMV proteins or antigens are being explored as potential immunotherapeutic agents to neutralize the virus, block entry into host cells, or enhance the immune response.

- **Immune checkpoint inhibitors:** These therapies aim to modulate the immune system's response by targeting immunosuppressive pathways, potentially enhancing the body's ability to recognize and eliminate CMV-infected cells.

Gene Therapy and Genetic Engineering:

Advances in gene therapy and genetic engineering technologies have opened up new possibilities for targeting and disrupting CMV infections at the molecular level. Approaches under investigation include:

- **Gene editing tools (CRISPR/Cas9):** These tools can potentially edit or disrupt viral genes or host cell factors crucial for viral replication, rendering the virus unable to propagate effectively.

- **RNA interference (RNAi):** This technology leverages small interfering RNA molecules to silence specific viral genes or cellular pathways involved in CMV replication and pathogenesis.

Combination Therapies:

The future of CMV treatment may involve the strategic combination of different therapeutic modalities, such as antiviral drugs, immunotherapies, and genetic interventions, to achieve synergistic effects and overcome drug resistance. Personalized medicine approaches, tailored to individual patient characteristics and viral strains, also play a role in optimizing treatment outcomes.

As research in these areas advances, the future of CMV treatment holds promise for more effective, targeted, and personalized approaches to managing this persistent viral infection. However, collaborative efforts among researchers, healthcare professionals, regulatory agencies, and industry partners will be crucial in translating these scientific discoveries.

Chapter 9

RESOURCES AND SUPPORT

Support Groups and Communities

Living with a cytomegalovirus (CMV) infection, whether as a patient, caregiver, or family member, can be a challenging journey filled with physical, emotional, and practical challenges. Support groups and communities can provide a valuable source of encouragement, understanding, and practical assistance for individuals navigating the complexities of CMV.

- **In-Person Support Groups:**
  Local in-person support groups, organized by healthcare facilities, non-profit organizations, or community centers, can offer a sense of

community and connection with others facing similar experiences. They can provide a safe space for sharing personal stories, exchanging coping strategies, and receiving emotional support from individuals who truly understand the challenges of living with CMV.

- **Online Support Communities:**
  In today's digital age, numerous online support communities have emerged, allowing individuals worldwide to connect and find support. These virtual communities may be forums, social media groups, or dedicated websites, providing a platform for individuals to share their experiences, ask questions, and receive guidance from others who have been through similar situations.

- **Disease-Specific Organizations:**
  Many non-profit organizations dedicated to specific diseases or conditions, such as congenital CMV or organ transplantation, offer support, resources, and programs for individuals affected by CMV. These organizations may provide educational

materials, host events or conferences, facilitate support group meetings, and advocate for research and awareness-raising efforts.

- **Peer Support Programs:**
Some healthcare facilities or organizations offer peer support programs that connect individuals living with CMV with trained volunteers or mentors who have personal experience navigating the challenges of the condition. These programs can provide one-on-one support, guidance, and a sense of shared understanding.

- **Caregiver Support:**
Caring for someone with a CMV infection can be physically and emotionally demanding. Support resources specifically designed for caregivers, such as respite care programs, counseling services, or caregiver support groups, can offer practical assistance, stress management tools, and a supportive community for those in caregiving roles.

- **Educational Resources:**
  In addition to emotional support, many organizations and healthcare providers offer educational resources, such as webinars, workshops, or informational materials, to help individuals and their families better understand CMV, its management, and the latest research and treatment developments.

Engaging with support groups and communities can provide a sense of empowerment, validation, and hope for individuals affected by CMV. By connecting with others who share similar experiences, individuals can access knowledge, practical advice, and emotional support, ultimately enhancing their ability to cope with CMV's challenges and improving their overall well-being.

Educational Materials and Outreach

Raising awareness and providing accurate, up-to-date information about cytomegalovirus (CMV) is crucial for promoting early detection, encouraging preventive measures, and supporting individuals affected by the infection. Educational materials and outreach efforts are vital in disseminating knowledge and fostering a better understanding of CMV among the general public, high-risk populations, and healthcare professionals.

- **Patient Education Materials:** Patient education materials, such as brochures, fact sheets, and multimedia resources, can provide individuals and families with accessible information about CMV, its transmission, symptoms, diagnosis, and treatment options. These materials should be written in clear, easy-to-understand language and tailored to various reading levels and cultural backgrounds.

- **Healthcare Professional Resources:** Healthcare professionals, including physicians, nurses, and specialists, require comprehensive and up-to-date resources to stay informed about the latest developments in CMV research, diagnostic methods, treatment guidelines, and best practices for patient care. Medical journals, clinical practice guidelines, and continuing education programs can be valuable resources for healthcare providers.

- **Public Awareness Campaigns:** Public awareness campaigns can play a crucial role in increasing knowledge about CMV, particularly among high-risk populations such as pregnant women, individuals with weakened immune systems, and healthcare workers. These campaigns may utilize various platforms, including social media, traditional media outlets, and community outreach events, to disseminate information and promote preventive measures.

- **Educational Seminars and Workshops:** Organizing educational seminars, workshops, or webinars can provide an interactive platform for individuals, caregivers, and healthcare professionals to learn about CMV from experts in the field. These events can cover many topics, such as symptom recognition, transmission prevention, treatment options, and coping strategies.

- **School and Daycare Education:** Educating staff and parents in schools, daycare centers, and other childcare settings about CMV can help raise awareness and promote preventive measures, as these environments are potential transmission sources. Educational materials and training programs can emphasize the importance of good hygiene practices, safe handling of bodily fluids, and recognizing potential signs of infection.

- **Collaboration with Patient Advocacy Groups:** Partnering with patient advocacy groups and non-profit organizations focused on CMV or related conditions can amplify educational outreach efforts. These organizations often have established networks, resources, and platforms to disseminate information and raise community awareness.

Effective educational materials and outreach efforts are essential for empowering individuals, caregivers, and healthcare professionals with the knowledge and tools necessary to navigate the challenges posed by CMV. By promoting awareness, providing accurate information, and fostering a better understanding of the infection, we can take proactive steps toward early detection, prevention, and improved management of CMV, ultimately enhancing the well-being of those affected by this persistent viral threat.

Advocacy and Policy Change

Advocacy and policy change are crucial in raising awareness, promoting research, and improving access to resources and support for individuals affected by cytomegalovirus (CMV) infections. By engaging in advocacy efforts and influencing policy decisions, various stakeholders can drive meaningful change and create a more supportive environment for those living with CMV.

- **Patient Advocacy Organizations:** Patient advocacy organizations, often led by individuals directly impacted by CMV or their caregivers, play a vital role in advocating for policy changes, increased funding for research, and improved access to healthcare and support services. These organizations can lobby policymakers, organize awareness campaigns, and amplify the voices of those affected by CMV.

- **Raising Awareness among Policymakers:** Advocacy efforts to raise awareness among policymakers and government officials are crucial for driving change. This can involve organizing advocacy events, scheduling meetings with elected representatives, and providing educational materials highlighting CMV's impact and the need for action.

- **Advocating for Increased Research Funding:** Advocating for increased funding for CMV research is essential for advancing scientific understanding, developing new diagnostic tools, and exploring novel treatment options and preventive strategies. Advocacy groups and stakeholders can work to ensure that CMV research remains a priority in both public and private funding initiatives.

- **Promoting Screening and Prevention Policies:** Advocacy efforts can focus on promoting policies that support screening and prevention programs for CMV, particularly for high-risk populations such as pregnant women and immunocompromised individuals. This may involve advocating for the inclusion of CMV screening in routine prenatal care or supporting the development and implementation of vaccination programs.

- **Improving Access to Healthcare and Support Services:** Advocating for improved access to healthcare and support services is crucial for ensuring that individuals affected by CMV can receive timely diagnosis, appropriate treatment, and the necessary support to manage the physical, emotional, and practical challenges associated with the infection.

- **Collaboration and Partnerships:** Building partnerships and collaborating with healthcare professionals, researchers, policymakers, and other stakeholders can amplify advocacy efforts and drive policy change more effectively. These collaborations can create a stronger voice and advocate for comprehensive solutions by leveraging collective expertise and resources.

Advocacy and policy change requires sustained efforts, perseverance, and a commitment to raising awareness and driving positive change. By engaging in advocacy initiatives, individuals, organizations, and stakeholders can create a more supportive and equitable environment for those affected by CMV, promote early detection, facilitate access to resources, and ultimately improve overall health outcomes.

Conclusion

Cytomegalovirus (CMV) is a widespread and persistent viral infection that challenges individuals, healthcare professionals, and society. While significant progress has been made in understanding and managing this complex virus, much work remains to overcome its obstacles and protect those most vulnerable to its potential consequences.

One of the primary challenges in conquering CMV is the need for greater awareness and knowledge about the infection among the general public and certain high-risk populations. Many individuals need to be more aware of the potential risks and impacts of CMV, which can lead to inadequate preventive measures, delayed diagnosis, and suboptimal management strategies. Raising public awareness through educational campaigns, robust outreach efforts, and comprehensive healthcare provider training is crucial to addressing this challenge.

Another significant hurdle is the limited availability of effective treatments and the emergence of drug resistance. While current antiviral medications have improved outcomes for many patients, their efficacy can be compromised by drug resistance or adverse side effects, especially in immunocompromised individuals. Continued investment in developing novel antiviral agents, immunotherapies, and genetic interventions is essential to providing more effective and targeted treatment options.

The absence of a licensed CMV vaccine further compounds the challenges of preventing and controlling the spread of the virus. Ongoing vaccine development efforts hold promise, but significant obstacles remain in producing a safe, effective, and widely accessible vaccine that can protect vulnerable populations, such as newborns, pregnant women, and immunocompromised individuals.

Addressing the long-term consequences of CMV infections, particularly in cases of congenital CMV or severe complications, is another critical challenge. Providing comprehensive support services, rehabilitation programs, and ongoing care for individuals affected by disabilities or chronic conditions resulting from CMV is essential to improving their quality of life and promoting optimal recovery.

Overcoming the challenges CMV poses requires a multifaceted approach involving collaboration among researchers, healthcare professionals, policymakers, patient advocacy groups, and the broader community. By fostering partnerships and leveraging collective expertise, resources, and advocacy efforts, we can drive advancements in prevention, diagnosis, treatment, and support for those affected by this persistent viral threat.

Ultimately, conquering CMV is not just a scientific or medical endeavor; it is a collective responsibility that requires a commitment to education, research, advocacy, and compassionate care. By addressing the challenges head-on and embracing a comprehensive approach, we can create a future where the impact of CMV is minimized, and those affected by the infection can live healthier, more fulfilling lives.

The Path Forward

Conquering the challenges posed by cytomegalovirus (CMV) requires a steadfast commitment to advancing scientific knowledge, fostering collaborative efforts, and implementing comprehensive strategies that address prevention, diagnosis, treatment, and support for those affected by this persistent viral infection.

The path forward must prioritize continued investment in research and development across multiple fronts. This includes:

- **Vaccine Development:** Accelerating efforts to develop safe and effective CMV vaccines that protect vulnerable populations, such as newborns, pregnant women, and immunocompromised individuals, remains a critical priority. Overcoming the scientific and logistical hurdles that have hindered previous vaccine development initiatives is crucial for achieving this goal.

- **Novel Antiviral Therapies:** Exploring new classes of antiviral compounds with unique mechanisms of action is essential to combat drug resistance and provide more effective treatment options for CMV infections. Collaboration between researchers, pharmaceutical companies, and regulatory agencies can expedite the translation of promising investigational agents into clinical practice.

- **Immunotherapeutic Approaches:** Harnessing the power of the immune system through strategies like CMV-specific T-cell therapies, monoclonal antibodies, and immune checkpoint inhibitors holds significant potential for enhancing the body's ability to fight CMV infections, particularly in immunocompromised individuals.

- **Genetic and Molecular Interventions:** Advances in gene therapy, genetic engineering, and molecular technologies open new avenues for targeting and disrupting CMV infections at the molecular level. Continued exploration of these cutting-edge approaches could lead to innovative treatment modalities and an improved understanding of host-virus interactions.

Alongside these research endeavors, robust public health initiatives and education campaigns are crucial for raising awareness, promoting preventive measures, and fostering early detection of CMV infections. Targeted outreach efforts should focus on high-risk populations, healthcare professionals, and the general public, utilizing various platforms and leveraging the expertise of patient advocacy groups and stakeholders.

Strengthening healthcare infrastructure and improving access to diagnostic testing, treatment, and supportive care services are also essential components of the path forward. This includes ensuring adequate resources for healthcare facilities, promoting best practices in CMV management, and providing comprehensive support services for individuals affected by the long-term consequences of CMV infections.

Furthermore, collaboration and partnerships among researchers, healthcare providers, policymakers, and patient advocacy groups must be fostered and sustained. By leveraging collective expertise, resources, and advocacy efforts, we can drive meaningful policy changes, secure funding for research and support services, and create a more equitable and supportive environment for those affected by CMV.

The path forward is undoubtedly challenging, but the potential rewards of conquering CMV are immense. By embracing a multifaceted approach that integrates scientific advancements, public health initiatives, healthcare infrastructure improvements, and collaborative efforts, we can pave the way for a future where the burden of CMV is significantly reduced. Those affected by this viral infection can live healthier, more fulfilling lives.

Appendices

Glossary of Terms

- **Antibody:** A protein produced by the immune system that recognizes and binds to specific antigens to help protect the body from harmful pathogens.
- **Antigen:** Any substance that causes the immune system to produce antibodies against it.
- **Asymptomatic:** Showing no symptoms of disease.
- **Congenital CMV:** Cytomegalovirus infection that occurs during pregnancy and is passed from mother to fetus.

- **Cytomegalovirus (CMV):** A common virus that can infect people of all ages and typically remains dormant in the body.
- **Immunocompromised:** Having an impaired or weakened immune system.
- **Latency:** The state in which a virus is present in the body but remains inactive or dormant.
- **Polymerase Chain Reaction (PCR):** A laboratory technique used to amplify and detect DNA and RNA sequences.
- **Seroprevalence:** The level of a pathogen in a population, as measured in blood serum.
- **Viremia:** The presence of viruses in the blood.

Frequently Asked Questions

1. ***What is Cytomegalovirus (CMV)?***
   CMV is a common virus that can infect people of all ages. Once infected, the virus remains in the body for life, typically in a dormant state.

2. ***How is CMV transmitted?***
   CMV is spread through close contact with body fluids, such as saliva, blood, urine, semen, and breast milk.

3. ***Who is at risk for CMV?***
   While anyone can contract CMV, it poses the highest risk to pregnant women, newborns, and individuals with weakened immune systems.

4. ***What are the symptoms of CMV?***
   Most people with CMV have no symptoms. However, when symptoms do occur, they can include fever, sore throat, fatigue, and swollen glands.

5. **How is CMV diagnosed?**

   CMV is diagnosed through laboratory tests, which can include blood tests, urine tests, and throat swabs.

6. **Can CMV be treated?**

   There is no cure for CMV, but antiviral medications can help control the virus and prevent or treat illness.

7. **Is there a vaccine for CMV?**

   Currently, there is no vaccine for CMV, but research is ongoing to develop one.

8. **Can CMV be prevented?**

   Good hygiene practices, such as handwashing, can help prevent the spread of CMV, especially for those at high risk.

9. **What complications can CMV cause?**

   In some cases, CMV can cause serious health problems, such as hearing loss, vision loss, and developmental disabilities, particularly in newborns.

10. ***Where can I find more information about CMV?***

Additional resources and support can be found in Chapter 9 of this book, as well as through healthcare providers and support organizations.

References and Further Reading

General CMV Information

- Mocarski, E. S., Shenk, T., Griffiths, P. D., & Pass, R. F. (2013). Cytomegalovirus. In *Fields Virology* (6th ed., Vol. 2, pp. 1960-2014). Lippincott Williams & Wilkins.
- Cannon, M. J., Schmid, D. S., & Hyde, T. B. (2010). Review of cytomegalovirus seroprevalence and demographic characteristics associated with infection. *Reviews in Medical Virology*, 20(4), 202-213.

Diagnosis and Laboratory Testing

- Lazzarotto, T., & Guerra, B. (2017). New advances in the diagnosis of congenital cytomegalovirus infection. *Journal of Clinical Virology*, 88, 19-24.
- Stagno, S., & Britt, W. J. (2012). Cytomegalovirus infections. In *Principles and Practice of Pediatric Infectious Diseases* (4th ed., pp. 1089-1097). Elsevier Saunders.

Treatment and Management

- Kimberlin, D. W., & Whitley, R. J. (2015). Antiviral therapy of HSV-1 and -2. In *Antiviral Research: Strategies in Antiviral Drug Discovery* (pp. 45-63). ASM Press.
- Griffiths, P. D., Stanton, A., McCarrell, E., Smith, C., Osman, M., Harber, M., ... & Emery, V. C. (2011). Cytomegalovirus glycoprotein-B vaccine with MF59 adjuvant in transplant recipients: a phase 2 randomised placebo-controlled trial. *The Lancet*, 377(9773), 1256-1263.

Prevention and Public Health

- Adler, S. P., & Marshall, B. (2007). Cytomegalovirus and child day care: Evidence for an increased infection rate among day-care workers. *The New England Journal of Medicine*, 317(10), 596-602.
- Pass, R. F., Zhang, C., Evans, A., Simpson, T., Andrews, W., Huang, M. L., ... & Britt, W. (2009). Vaccine prevention of maternal cytomegalovirus infection. *The New England Journal of Medicine*, 360(12), 1191-1199.

www.ingramcontent.com/pod-product-compliance
Lightning Source LLC
Chambersburg PA
CBHW070806260726
48660CB00005B/1723